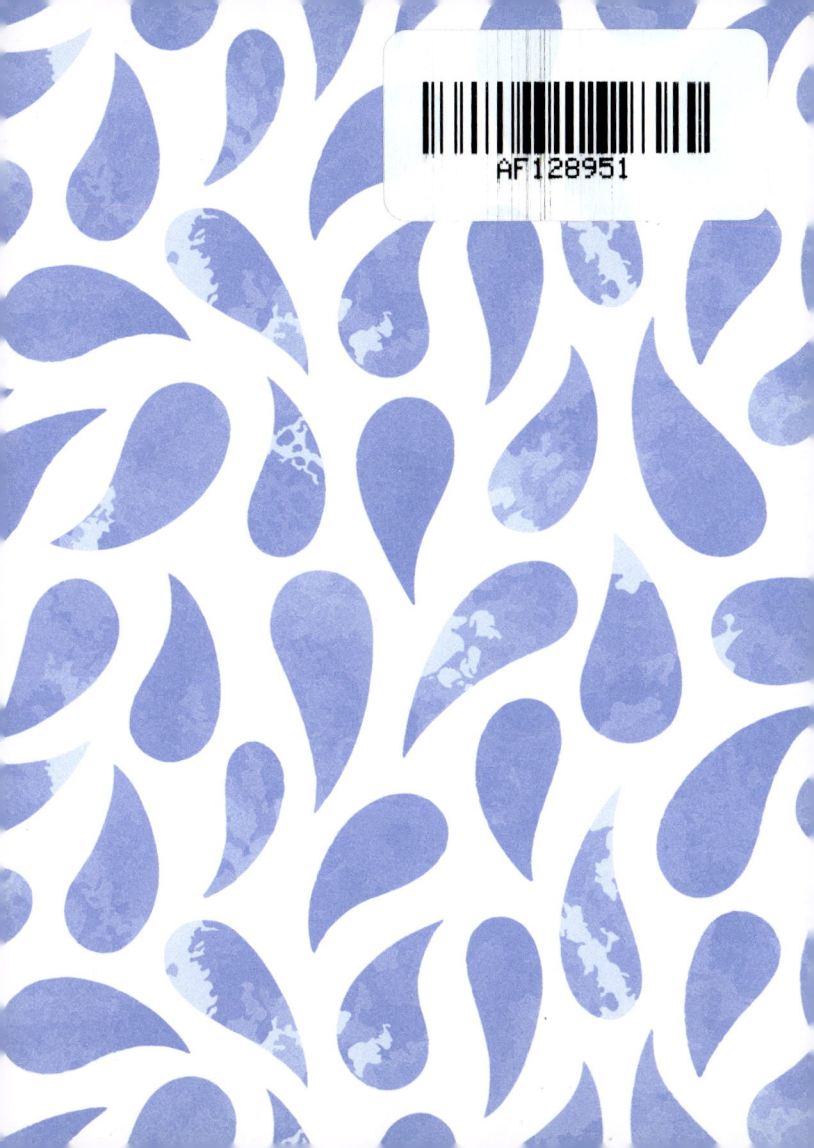

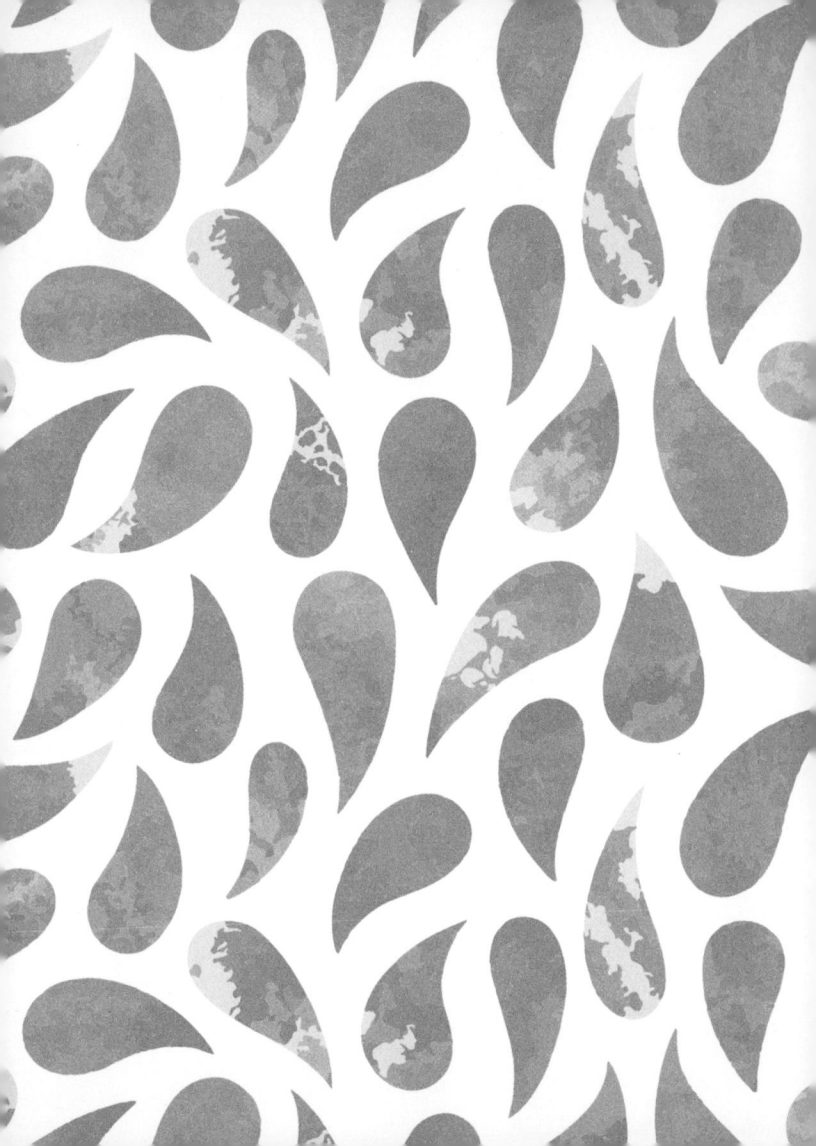

The
A–Z
of
Longevity

THE A–Z OF LONGEVITY

Copyright © Octopus Publishing Group Limited, 2026

All rights reserved.

Text by Jennifer Cordero

No part of this book may be reproduced by any means, nor transmitted, nor translated into a machine language, without the written permission of the publishers.

Condition of Sale
This book is sold subject to the condition that it shall not, by way of trade or otherwise, be lent, resold, hired out or otherwise circulated in any form of binding or cover other than that in which it is published and without a similar condition including this condition being imposed on the subsequent purchaser.

An Hachette UK Company
www.hachette.co.uk

Vie Books, an imprint of Summersdale Publishers
Part of Octopus Publishing Group Limited
Carmelite House
50 Victoria Embankment
LONDON
EC4Y 0DZ
UK

This FSC® label means that materials and other controlled sources used for the product have been responsibly sourced

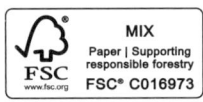

www.summersdale.com

The authorized representative in the EEA is Hachette Ireland, 8 Castlecourt Centre, Dublin 15, D15 XTP3, Ireland (email: info@hbgi.ie)

Printed and bound in China

ISBN: 978-1-83799-775-6
eISBN: 978-1-83799-776-3

Substantial discounts on bulk quantities of Summersdale books are available to corporations, professional associations and other organizations. For details contact general enquiries: telephone: +44 (0) 1243 771107 or email: enquiries@summersdale.com.

Neither the author nor the publisher can be held responsible for any injury, loss or claim – be it health, financial or otherwise – arising out of the use, or misuse, of the suggestions made herein. This book is not intended as a substitute for the medical advice of a doctor or physician. If you are experiencing problems with your physical or mental health, it is always best to follow the advice of a medical professional.

The A–Z of Longevity

How to Live a Longer, Healthier Life

Anna Barnes

Introduction

Welcome to *The A–Z of Longevity*, a thoughtful guide designed to help you explore the art and science of living well for longer. In a world often focused on speed and productivity, the idea of lasting vitality can sometimes feel elusive. But longevity isn't just about adding years to your life – it's about adding life to those years. This book offers a gentle, practical approach to embracing habits that nurture body, mind and spirit across the decades.

Drawing on ancient wisdom and modern scientific studies, *The A–Z of Longevity* guides you through simple, effective strategies for healthy ageing. Each letter highlights a key element of well-being – from movement and mindfulness, to nutrition and connection – presented in accessible, bite-sized insights you can return to time and again.

Whether you're just beginning to consider your long-term health or are seeking to refine the path you're already on, this book meets you where you are. You'll find ideas to inspire action, activities that spark reflection and tips to take into your everyday life.

As you turn the pages, may you feel empowered to make small, sustainable choices that lead to a longer, fuller life. See this as your invitation to slow down, check in and embrace practices that support a vibrant future – one letter and one moment at a time.

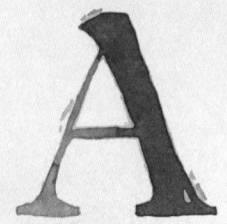

is for
Attitude

Good news for the optimists out there: it turns out that looking on the bright side of life contributes to healthy ageing! In fact, optimists might live 11 to 15 per cent longer than their pessimistic pals, due to their more frequent engagement with age-positive healthy habits.

A positive mental attitude isn't just about smiling through it all, though. It's about understanding that life will have its ups and downs, but we each have a choice in how we respond to these natural ebbs and flows. Where optimists will see obstacles as something to be overcome in pursuit of their goals, pessimists might lack the confidence to continue, giving up before achieving their desired outcome. These two diverging attitudes can have a strong ripple effect, influencing our health, relationships and overall outlook on life.

Scientifically speaking, there are positive correlations that show optimism might be an effective tool for slowing down cellular ageing. But don't worry, you don't have to be a born optimist – you can learn to change your ways. Only about 25 per cent of the population are born with sunny dispositions. Like a muscle, optimism can be strengthened with time and effort. Nurturing a more optimistic outlook can build resilience and help you better manage stress. That's good news, isn't it?

The "best possible self" exercise is widely recognized as an effective tool for boosting optimism, as well as increasing levels of hope and positivity. Visualization and imagination can be powerful tools to utilize in your quest to become more optimistic. Try this over the course of two weeks – you might be pleasantly surprised with the results.

1. Grab a notebook and pen.
2. Find a quiet place where you won't be disturbed for 10 to 15 minutes.
3. Pick a date in the future, perhaps in a few years' time, but no more than five.
4. Close your eyes and imagine the best possible life for yourself at this future date.
5. Consider all aspects of your life: relationships, health, career, studies, hobbies.
6. Add as much detail to the visualization as you can.
7. Open your eyes and start free-writing continuously about this best possible future.

Dos and don'ts

- 💧 Do be specific: include detailed descriptions for everything you write.
- 💧 Don't be tempted to edit your imagination.
- 💧 Do write without restriction – this isn't the time for planning or practicality.
- 💧 Don't worry about grammar or spelling.

Once you're done, keep the paper somewhere safe so that you can return to it over the next two weeks. Take time, ideally 10 to 15 minutes each day, to review your "best possible self" visualization and engage with the details of what this life looks like.

> You only live once, but if you do it right, once is enough.
>
> Mae West

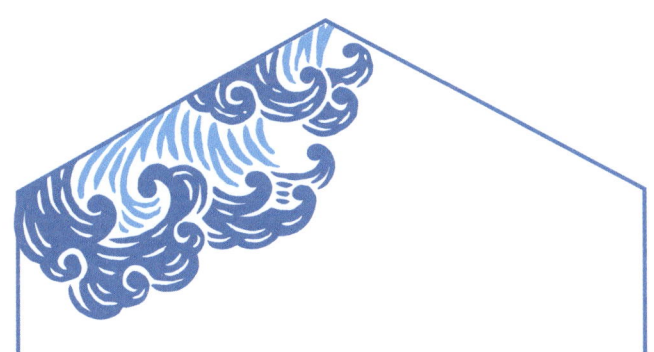

Everything you think, say and do can make you healthier

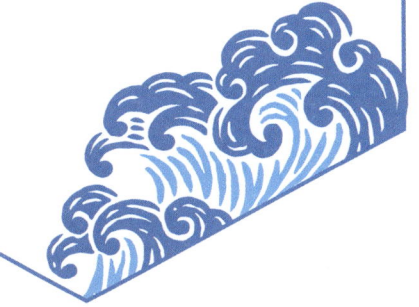

B

is for
Balance

The ability to balance on one leg might be the best indicator of longevity. Balance is tied to so many critical body functions that any decline in this area is a clear warning sign. Consider this: every step you take is a controlled falling motion. Thankfully, your brain can coordinate the necessary inputs from multiple systems in the body, to ensure you stay upright with each potential tumble.

Balance requires our brains to register the fluid in our ear canals, our eyes to provide visual guidance and our nervous system to provide proprioception information on our place in space. This then feeds back to our muscles to direct the movement, and finally our cardiovascular system feeds in, to ensure enough oxygen is being fed into the body. With any weak links in this chain, our balance can become compromised. No wonder it's a key indicator of our biological ageing.

Though our natural ability to balance starts to decline from mid-life, maintaining an active lifestyle can mitigate the level of deterioration. Dynamic balance exercises, including the following, are the most effective type for improving balance:

- Taking the stairs rather than the lift.
- Walking just on your toes or heels.
- Balancing on one leg (with appropriate safety support if necessary).
- Practising yoga.
- Dancing.

People who are good at multi-tasking have fewer falls. This capacity can start to decline in adults as young as 30. Enhancing the mind–body connection is vital to maintaining healthy balance. Here are a few cognitive loading exercises, to challenge your balance and brain at the same time:

- Try standing on one leg and counting backwards from 100 in sevens.
- Swap legs and count to 100 in sixes.
- Walk forwards in a straight line, heel-to-toe, reciting the months of the year in reverse from December.
- Walk backwards in a straight line, toe-to-heel, reciting the days of the week in reverse order.

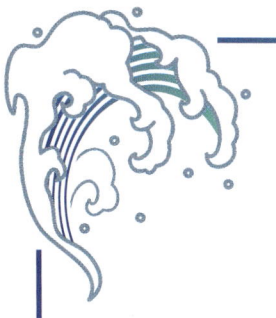

Your power comes from your choices. No one can stop you but yourself.

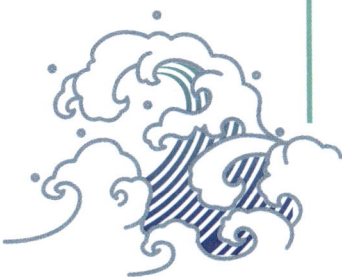

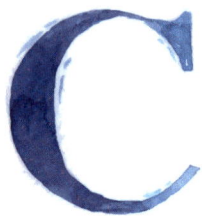

is for
Connection

Want to live a long and happy life? The good news is, you're much more likely to do that if you do it with friends. Our relationships with others are the single most significant factor in determining overall happiness – and happy people are proven to live longer. Strong social ties and solid emotional connections can offer support during hard times and amplify our good humour during joyful times.

Studies have shown that the negative impact of social isolation and loneliness is equivalent to that of physical inactivity, obesity and smoking, and can lead to a 25 per cent greater risk of early death.

On the plus side, strong connections and healthy relationships lead to reduced stress, lower blood pressure and increased levels of happiness – all great markers for a long and healthy life. Put simply, strong relationships can help you live longer. Longevity researchers are starting to rank social fitness as equally important as physical fitness... maybe it's time to phone a friend and share this news with them!

Top tip
As we get older, our social lives may dwindle. Finding time to socialize on top of all the other things on our to-do lists can be a challenge. One way to combat this is to combine activities. So, offer to help your friend with their gardening, or the next time you're going for a walk, invite a friend along. You'll reap double the rewards – both physical and social fitness.

Volunteering is a great way to meet new people while helping support your local community – and perhaps even learning a new skill, too. Keep an eye out in local newspapers and online for organizations needing help, or contact your local community centre. Whether it's supporting a one-off activity or event, or becoming a regular volunteer, you'll benefit from an increased sense of purpose while lending support to a worthy cause.

The following actively encourage volunteers:

- Animal shelters
- Libraries
- Community planting projects
- Museums and art galleries
- Local attractions

Perhaps the secret of living well is not in having all the answers but in pursuing unanswerable questions in good company.

Rachel Naomi Remen

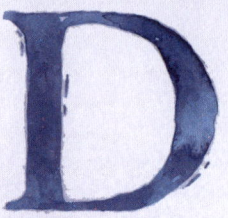

is for
Diet

A balanced diet is not just key to living a long and healthy life – it's the way to do it deliciously! Eating the rainbow is an easy way to incorporate more variety and a wider range of vitamins, minerals and essential nutrients into your life. Aim to cover all the colours in a day and change up your choices to keep your tastebuds tingling.

Here's some inspiration to get you started:

- Red: tomatoes, red peppers, watermelon, strawberries, red cabbage and cherries.
- Orange: carrots, sweet potatoes, butternut squash, mangoes, oranges and apricots.
- Yellow: sweetcorn, yellow courgettes, bananas, lemons, pineapples and yellow bell peppers.
- Green: broccoli, spinach, avocado, asparagus, kiwi, green beans, celery, lettuce and limes.
- Purple: blueberries, blackberries, aubergines, red onions, beetroot and grapes.

The beautiful thing about eating a broad rainbow diet is there's no need for calorie counting or eliminating any particular type of food. Love chocolate? No problem – eaten in moderation, it can form part of a healthy diet. Keep in mind the 70/20/10 rule, where you aim to get 70 per cent of your calories from fruits, vegetables and grains, 20 per cent from lean protein, such as chicken, fish, lentils or beans, and 10 per cent from fats.

Keep a food diary to track your rainbow progress. Each week, write down the foods you ate in each of the colours. At the end of a month, you'll start to see which areas need a boost and which are on track.

List the red food items you ate this week:

....

....

List the orange food items you ate this week:

....

....

List the yellow food items you ate this week:

....

....

List the green food items you ate this week:

....

....

List the purple food items you ate this week:

....

....

One cannot think well,

love well, sleep well,

if one has not dined well.

Virginia Woolf

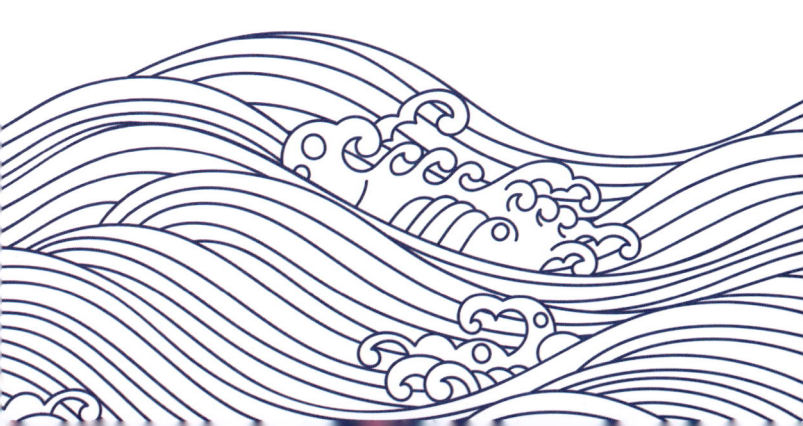

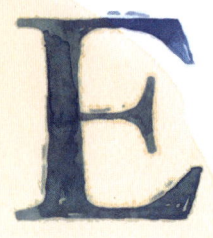

is for
Exercise

A daily dose of exercise is recommended for anyone wanting to add quality of life to their later years. In fact, the earlier you start incorporating regular exercise into your routine, the more benefits you will reap. Studies have confirmed that adults who engage in 150 minutes per week of moderate exercise (think a brisk walk) or 75 minutes of more vigorous exercise (such as running) cut their risk of early death by one third.

Regularly getting your heart pumping faster has a dramatic impact on longevity and decreases risk factors associated with heart disease, cancer, diabetes and cognitive decline.

Wondering which exercise is most effective for improving your overall health and well-being? Experts recommend dividing your efforts evenly into cardio and weight-bearing activities. Not the gym type? No problem. By increasing your everyday activity levels, you can make movement a part of your life. Walking, yoga, dancing and tai chi can all be done with relative ease and without much extra equipment or a trip to the gym. Ultimately, the best exercise for you is the one you enjoy the most. Then it's a choice, rather than a chore.

Top tip

Try decreasing your inactive times. "Movement snacks" are small bouts of activity that reduce long periods of sitting. Practise a few squats while waiting for the kettle to boil, march on the spot while brushing your teeth, or park your car in the spot furthest away in the car park from your destination.

Make a SMART exercise goal. SMART goals are specific, measurable, achievable, relevant and time-bound.

S: What is my goal? Why is it important to me?

....

....

M: How will I measure success? How will I know I've achieved my goal?

....

....

A: What steps will I take to achieve this goal? How will I hold myself accountable?

....

....

R: How does this goal fit my vision for my future? How does it align with my values?

....

....

T: When will I accomplish my goal? How long will I need to reach this achievement?

....

....

Steps to achieving my goal

Description	Time estimate	Completion date

Obstacles that may arise	How I will respond

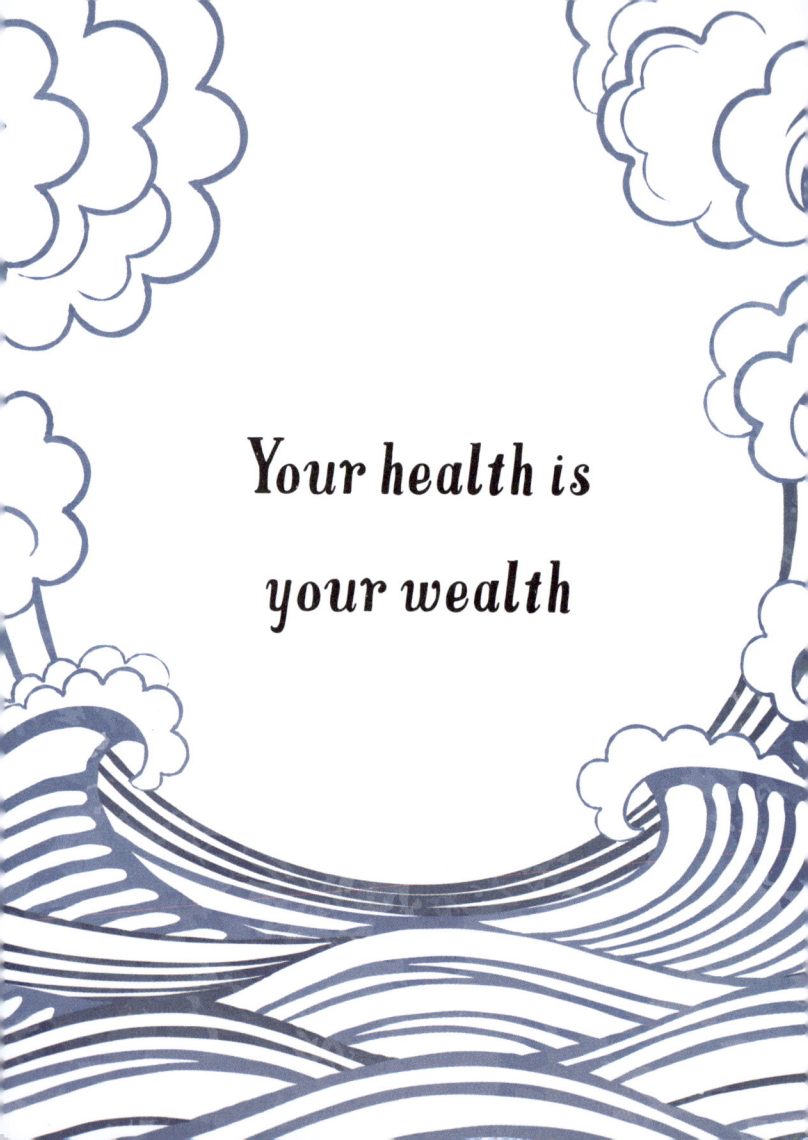

If you don't make time

for exercise, you'll probably

have to make time for illness.

Robin Sharma

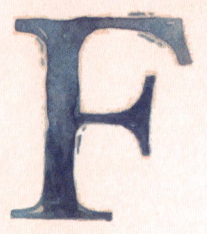

is for
Fun

In 1959, Kim Knor took her first jump out of a plane and fell in love with skydiving. Sixty-six years later, aged 86, she started travelling around the US totting up jumps with the aim of reaching 1,000. The spritely octogenarian is a great reminder that life is a journey and we should all enjoy the ride.

Think fun is frivolous? Think again. Having fun isn't just for kids – adults benefit from play as much as children. Engaging in fun activities is a stress reliever and encourages connection with others. It stimulates imagination, encourages problem-solving and even helps in forming friendships. Engaging in activities that bring joy, fulfilment and satisfaction can bring us into a "flow" state, which strengthens our mental well-being, meaning that playful adults are better able to cope in stressful situations.

Try to recall the activities you enjoyed as a child. Did you love drawing? Sports? Building things? How can you incorporate these activities into your everyday life?

Making time for fun is easier than you might think. You can schedule fun time into your calendar. Seek out people who make you laugh, watch funny shows or listen to funny podcasts. Don't be afraid of looking silly – the world is serious enough. We can all use another reason to smile.

Learn to hula hoop. Not only is it fun, but it also improves cardiovascular fitness, balance, coordination and core strength.

To get started:

1. Stand normally and place one foot forwards.
2. Hold the hula hoop at waist level, touching your back, with the hoop parallel to the floor.
3. Start circling your hips around right to left.
4. When you're ready, release the hoop in a circular motion and keep moving your hips around.

Don't be discouraged if it takes a while to get the hang of it. At least you'll be smiling the whole time!

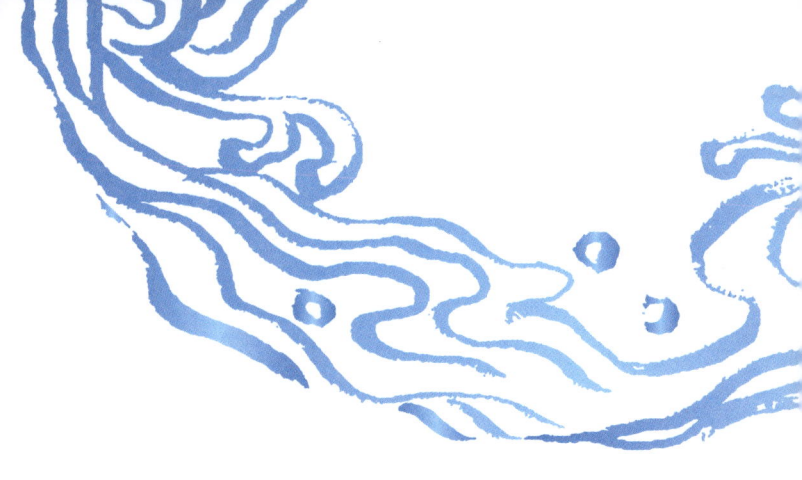

We don't stop playing

because we grow old;

we grow old because

we stop playing.

George Bernard Shaw

is for
Gardening

There's no better place to plant the seeds of longevity than in your very own garden. Studies of the world's five "blue zones", where locals are known for their longevity, revealed an interesting connection. In each of these areas, gardening was an activity enjoyed by adults well into their eighties and even nineties. Not only do gardeners live longer, they're also less stressed and have a lower risk of dementia than their non-planting pals.

Outdoor exercise – even gentle pottering around in the garden – can boost mood and improve social connection. In Okinawa, a famed blue zone, residents believe everyone needs an *ikigai*, or reason for living, to grow old healthfully. A garden offers that perfect combination of responsibility and reward.

Incredibly, studies have shown that even looking at a garden can have tangible benefits. But don't let that stop you from digging in – some of the greatest health benefits from gardening happen by getting your hands dirty. Soil is rich in beneficial bacteria that can help in the fight against allergies and inflammatory diseases.

Finally, gardening can bring an immense sense of achievement. Nurturing seeds, watching them spring from the ground and grow over time – perhaps producing beautiful flowers or tasty fruit or veg – is immensely satisfying.

With all the benefits of gardening that await, maybe it's time to get planting.

Start a garden today. There's no need to wait until springtime to get growing – gardening is a year-round activity. Look online or in your local library for a 12-month seasonal guide. No outdoor space? No problem – indoor pots are a great way to get your green fix.

Here are some beginner-friendly plants to get you started:

Flowers
- Impatiens
- Lavender
- Marigolds
- Morning Glories
- Pansies
- Sunflowers
- Zinnias

Fruit and vegetables
- Beetroot
- Chillies
- Courgettes/zucchini
- Potatoes (can even be grown in pots!)
- Shallots
- Squashes
- Strawberries

To plant
a garden
is to believe
in tomorrow.

Audrey Hepburn

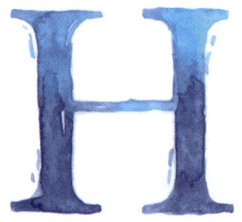

is for
Hugs

The best things in life are free and hugs are right up there on the list. A hug can convey so many emotions, from comfort to excitement. Hugs release oxytocin into our system and increase our serotonin levels, both of which counteract cortisol production. Think of hugs as your triple whammy of hormone balancing that impacts mood, reduces stress and improves overall well-being.

Hugs have a direct impact on stress. One study showed a link between regular huggers and lower blood pressure and heart rate when faced with stressful events. Hugs have also been found to help fight off the common cold. Wrapping your arms around someone, or having their arms wrapped around you, is such a powerful gesture that it can even help reduce levels of anxiety and fear. Our feeling of safety and belonging is increased with every embrace.

If you're not a natural hugger, don't worry. For some, holding hands can offer similar benefits. And hugging doesn't have to be only between humans to have a positive impact – cuddling a pet or even a favourite teddy bear can provide that powerful feeling of comfort and sensation of touch.

How many hugs are needed to reap the benefits? One expert shared that four hugs per day are necessary for survival, eight for maintenance and twelve for growth. Why not share this thought with someone you love over a hug?

Inspired by zen master Thích Nhất Hạnh, this hugging meditation can be practised with a partner, friend or even a tree.

1. Start by bowing, to recognize the other's presence.
2. Take three deep breaths to root yourself.
3. Open your arms to embrace the other for three more breaths. With the first, become aware of the present moment, feeling happiness. With the second, become aware of the other being present in the moment, feeling happiness. With the final breath, feel the presence of both of you, together, at this moment in time, offering gratitude and happiness for your togetherness.

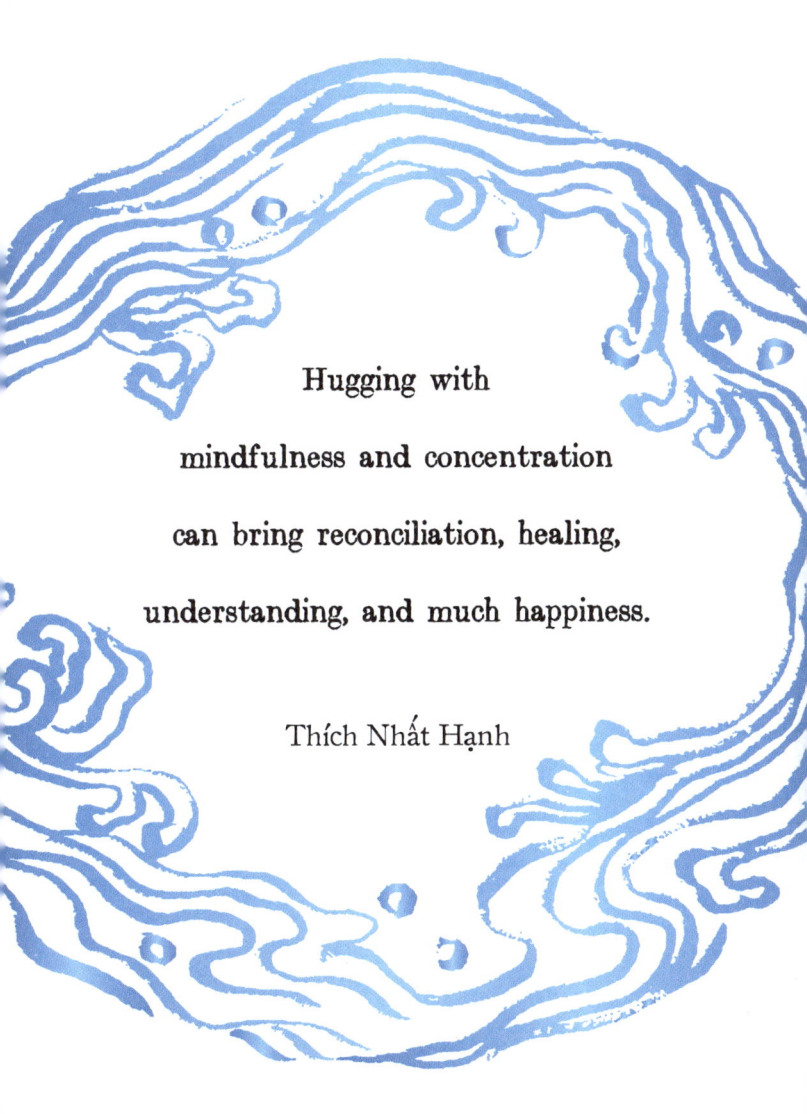

Hugging with

mindfulness and concentration

can bring reconciliation, healing,

understanding, and much happiness.

Thích Nhất Hạnh

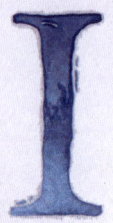

is for
Imagination

Do you ever wonder why children are encouraged to use their imaginations? Flexing our imagination is a form of cognitive development that builds emotional capacity. As we get older, we're encouraged to think more logically than creatively, causing a decline in our imagination. But there's good reason for unearthing our imagination as we age.

Imagination is a powerful tool that can improve your present, shape your future and even help mend your past. It can fuel passion and motivation, and spark creativity at any age – and there's nothing quite like a new-found interest to energize your day. Engaging in imaginative activities is a stress-buster, too – even simple daydreaming can lower cortisol levels. Imagination can provide a path to a better future, helping us move past difficult situations.

A strong imagination also acts as an aide memoire to preserve your memories. Using your imagination creates more neurons in the brain and reduces the likelihood of developing memory problems that can lead to dementia.

What's more, the ability to imagine your own future is a strong incentive for developing healthy habits at a young age. The more vividly you can connect to your future self, the more likely you are to want to take steps today to ensure you can be the best version of yourself as you age.

Imagination is improved with practice, so try the 30 circles exercise.

Set a timer for 3 minutes, and grab some coloured pencils or markers. Start the timer, then try to turn the circles into recognizable objects – beach ball, ladybug, eyeball etc. See how many you can finish in 3 minutes. Repeat the exercise over the next few weeks and compare any differences.

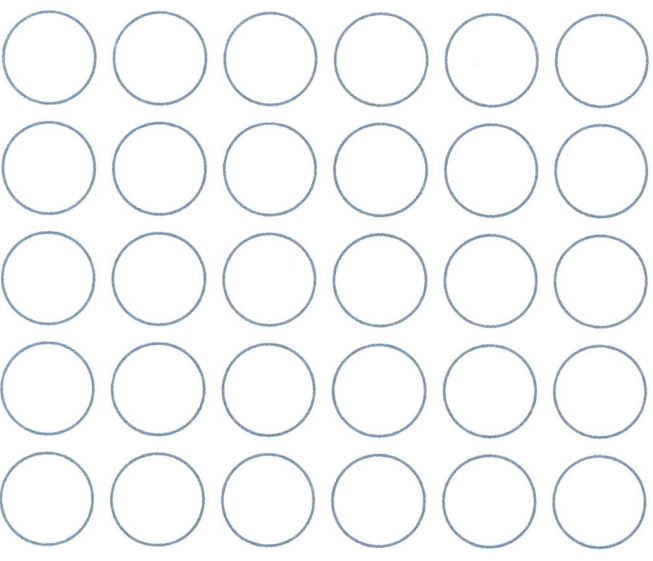

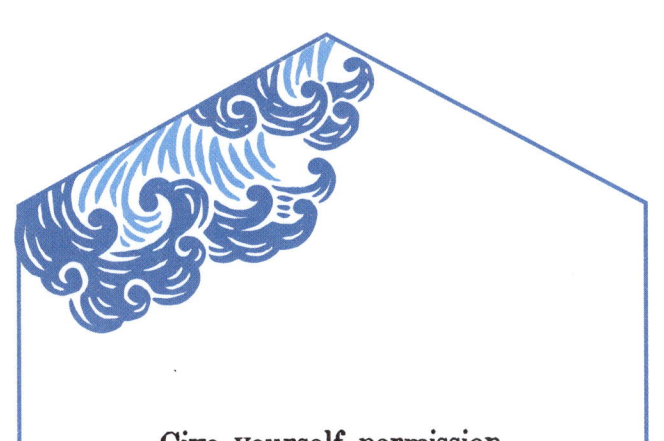

Give yourself permission

to imagine freely

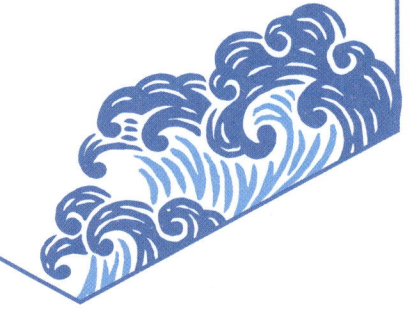

J is for *Joy*

Joy is a deep sense of satisfaction and contentment. It surpasses feelings of happiness, which can be fleeting. While happiness is something we might pursue, joy is an expansive emotion that can influence our outlook on life. For example, we might feel happy that we are able to catch up with an old friend we've not seen for a while; whereas joy rests in the bonds of that friendship forged over years of shared experience.

Experiencing joy has a positive impact on the physical body. Breathing accelerates, the heart rate quickens and even body temperature can increase, all due to an adrenaline boost. The physiological changes associated with joy can trigger activity in pleasure-related hot spots in the brain, so feeling joyful actually initiates more joy. Joyful people are more likely to engage in other healthy activities, such as healthy eating, exercise and balanced sleep – key factors to foster longevity.

Moreover, the genuine smile that joy induces has a range of health benefits. The Duchenne smile, an involuntary smile that reaches our eyes, improves physical health and connection with others, and can even help boost recovery after illness.

While joy might seem more elusive than happiness, it's actually easy to find joy by looking for it in the little things. A beautiful sunset, the sound of rain and the smell of freshly cut grass are all things that can bring a sense of deep joy.

Keeping a joy jar is a great way to help you focus on the joy in your life.

Find a large glass jar you can keep on your desk or somewhere that means you'll see it regularly. At the end of each day, take a piece of paper and write down something that brought you joy, along with the date. Fold it up and pop it in the jar. As the jar fills, it will remind you how much joy there is in your life and encourage you to keep looking for joy around you.

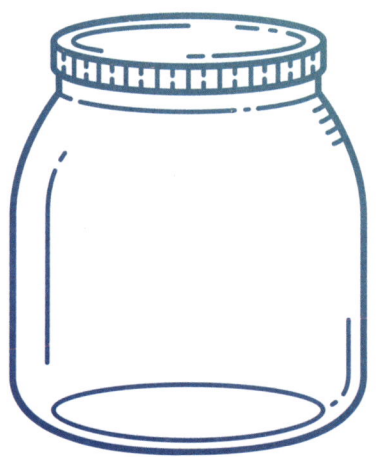

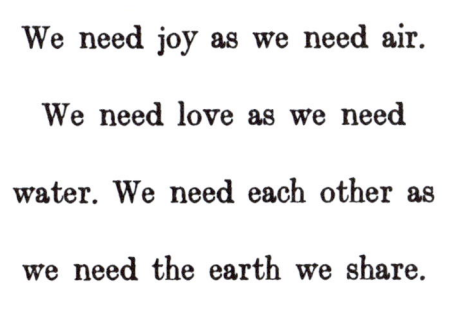

We need joy as we need air. We need love as we need water. We need each other as we need the earth we share.

Maya Angelou

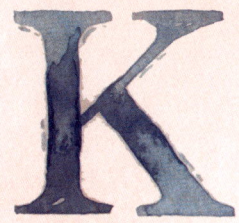

is for
Kaizen

Kaizen is a Japanese concept that broadly translates as "continuous improvement". The idea is that small and steady movement in the right direction is easiest to maintain and most effective long-term. Oftentimes, when faced with concerns about health and well-being, the human instinct is to go big and get there fast. Sweeping changes are planned. Restrictive eating, regimented exercise and other hard-to-maintain goals are put in place, with the hope of overnight improvement. Sadly, these "all or nothing" regimens often end in disappointment and disillusionment.

The *Kaizen* approach advocates embracing small, consistent efforts towards improvement, recognizing that transformation is a process, not just an activity. By adopting the slow and steady approach, healthier habits become ingrained as they are repeated and turn into gradual lifestyle changes. Over time, these small changes add up to big results. In fact, we can rewire our brain through repetition, forming positive habits and fuelling personal growth.

Kaizen also encourages us to think more long-term about the continuity of action and impact. We see that how we choose to live today has a direct impact on who we become in the future. Choosing to embrace this understanding can motivate healthier decision-making and pave the way for a happier, healthier tomorrow.

Sometimes, we get so focused on eliminating our bad habits or working on our weaknesses that we forget we're very likely already doing lots of good things, too. Try choosing one area of your life that you'd like to improve and commit to building on your existing good actions. For example, if you want to become more physically fit and you love walking, then commit to a 10-minute walk after dinner every evening.

Area you'd like to improve:

....

Good habits you already follow:

....

....

....

How can you amplify these habits daily?

....

....

....

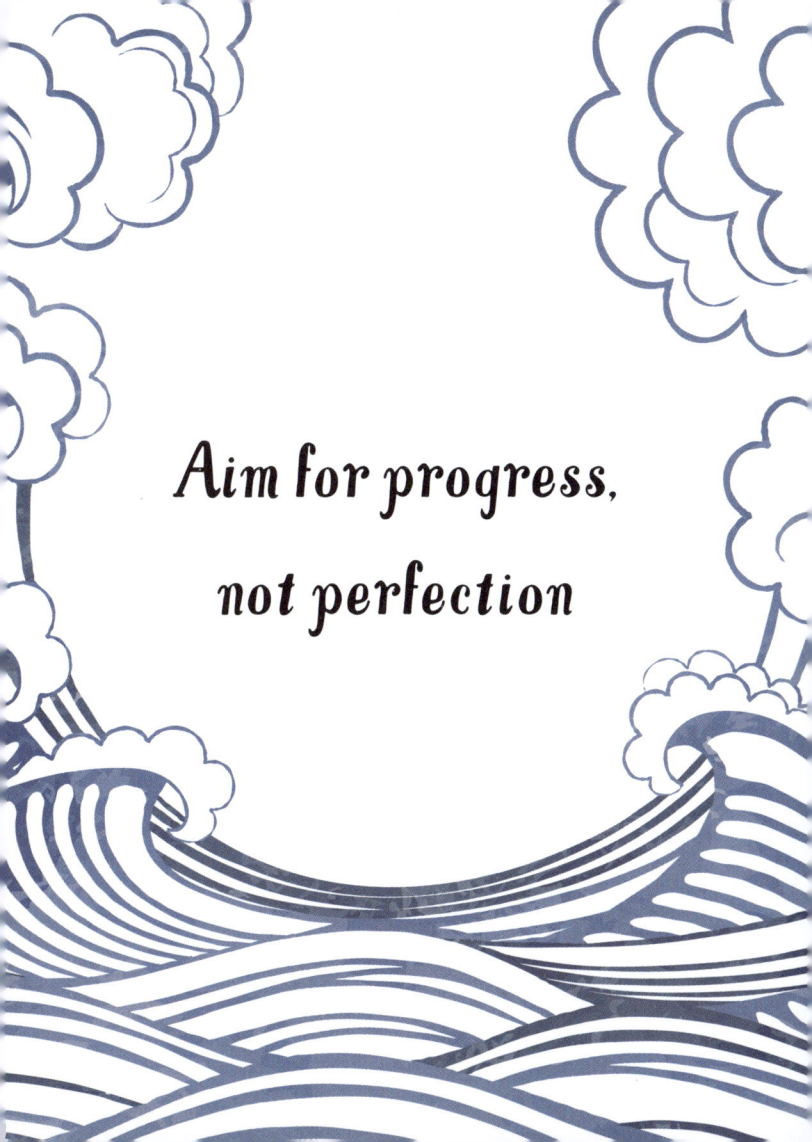

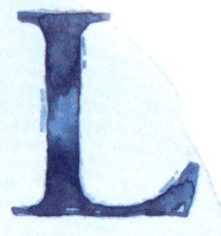

L

is for
Learning

Do you aim to learn something new every day? If so, you're not just getting smarter, you're reaping a whole host of other benefits as well. Learning keeps you young. Science proves that our brains continue to adapt to new experiences, regardless of age. When we try something new or learn a new skill, our brains create neural pathways that develop our resilience and build self-esteem.

Lifelong learners are more optimistic and less stressed. They have sharper cognitive abilities, even as they age. Learning new things can also assist in warding off dementia and Alzheimer's disease. When it comes to our brain's capacity to create new neural connections, it's a case of use it or lose it. Our ability doesn't fade with age; it fizzles out through lack of engagement. New research suggests seniors who learn multiple new things could shave years off their brain age, keeping age-related illnesses at bay. So, instead of just dutifully finishing your daily crossword, experiment with new types of puzzles and activities, to challenge your cognitive abilities.

It takes as little as 2 hours a week of active learning to combat mental decline. That doesn't mean you have to bury your nose in a book for those 2 hours – there are opportunities all around us to learn new skills and gain knowledge. Learning a new sport, figuring out how to use different functions on your mobile device or dusting off the chessboard for a match are all great ways to flex your grey matter.

Tracking your learning in a journal is a powerful way to reinforce your new skills, while also providing a tactile and visual reminder of your progress. Putting pen to paper is a transformative step in learning. Hence, even the simple act of writing can fire up a series of cognitive processes in multiple areas of the brain. This facilitates the processing of information and ideas, meaning you're more likely to understand and retain information if you write it down.

Take time to create your perfect learning journal. Look for a special notebook – think about its size and the texture of the paper, and personalize the cover with your own images or words in a collage. You could even buy a special pen that you only use for your journal. Keep your learning journal strictly on topic, and consider purchasing a new journal for each year.

Things to keep in mind when you're starting a learning journal for yourself:

- Try updating your learning journal regularly, even if some days the entries are short.
- Focus on a specific topic for individual entries. Think about how you can address those issues, then focus on how those issues can be resolved or improved.
- Look up questions or prompts on that topic, to help you focus on your learning journey more effectively.
- Avoid any kind of descriptive writing in your journal – concentrate instead on logical reasoning.
- At the end of each month, review your entries and try to identify any common themes. Focus on recognizing any long-term action you might need to take on those specific learning topics.

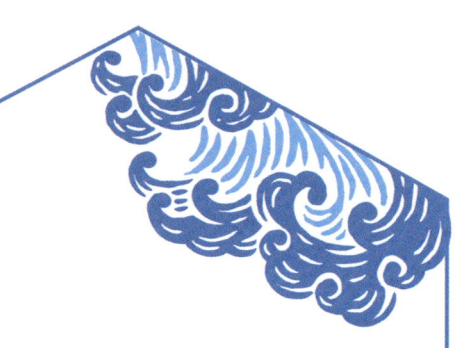

Every day is a new day

to learn and grow

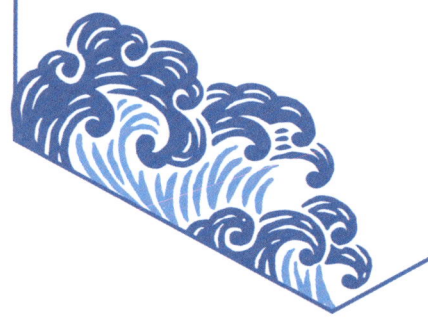

There is no one more foolish

than one who stops learning.

Seneca

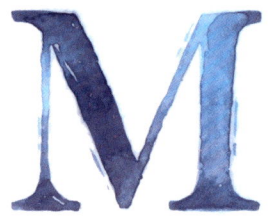

is for
Music

Listening to or playing music is like taking your mind to the gym for a workout. The way the brain interacts with music is unlike any other engagement – and studies show it's not just unique, but it also slows cognitive decline as we age. In a fascinating study, participants were given weekly piano lessons and practised five days a week. This not only increased the grey matter in four areas of their brains, including working memory, but they also maintained matter in a fifth area of the brain, where the non-piano players showed decline.

Music can elevate your mood and stimulate positive feelings. When you listen to music, neurotransmitters such as dopamine and endorphins are released that act as natural painkillers. Listening to music while you're suffering can reduce the intensity of the pain.

Our brains form a bond with the music we listen to when we're young, and studies have shown that listening to that music when we're older can have a counterclockwise, anti-ageing effect. When we hear music from our past, it activates multiple parts of the brain, and can even release dopamine and serotonin into our systems.

Music also increases energy levels and alertness, through increased blood flow to our extremities. So, whether you prefer rock, pop, classical or jazz, there's good reason to tune in and turn up the volume.

Expand your taste in tunes, to keep your musical mind active.

What genres of music do you naturally gravitate towards?

....
....
....

What genres are you interested in exploring further?

....
....
....

Ask family and friends to swap playlists with you, then note any songs and/or artists you discover. Use this space to write down how this new music makes you feel.

....
....
....
....

Music is the soundtrack of our individual lives.

Dick Clark

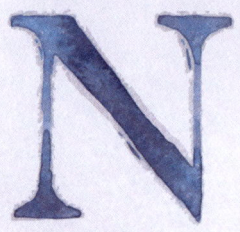

is for
Nature

If you're hoping to add some colour to your later years, your best bet is to go green. Time spent in nature can soothe the soul and quieten the mind. Not only does this help restore better balance to our biological selves, but it might also have a direct impact on our longevity. Studies have shown that the risk of death by heart disease and stroke is reduced by living in areas with more green vegetation, in part due to the lower pollution levels. In one study, risk of serious respiratory disease was cut by one third in women who lived near the highest amount of vegetation.

Urbanites can also reap the benefits of nature, by visiting green spaces in their local environment. Spending at least 2 hours a week in nature has been shown to significantly improve overall health and well-being. In fact, city dwellers who take regular green breaks are less likely to need medication for anxiety, depression and asthma. So, try to trade the urban jungle for some gentle greener pastures for a few hours each week.

Green space has a further plus point, in that it encourages exercise. Whether they are walking, gardening or taking their favourite four-legged friend out for a jaunt, people living near greenery experience less of a decline in physical activity as they age.

Get to know your neighbours! Our communities are not just made up of people, but also the other living things that surround us. When you're out and about on a walk, look for plants or animals you don't recognize. Use the space below to note down any that are unfamiliar to you, then look them up to learn more.

List your local...

Animals:

....
....
....

Birds:

....
....
....

Trees:

....
....
....

Plants and shrubs:

....
....
....

Flowers:

....
....
....

Insects:

....
....
....

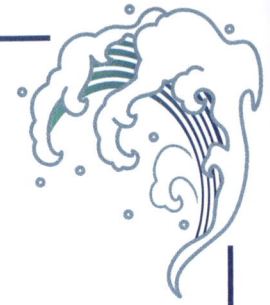

I live in harmony with the natural world around me

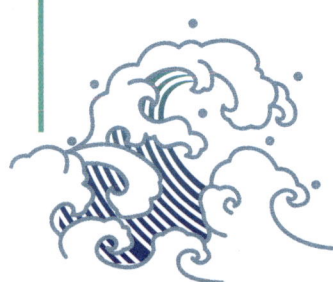

Live in the sunshine,

swim the sea,

drink the wild air's salubrity.

Ralph Waldo Emerson

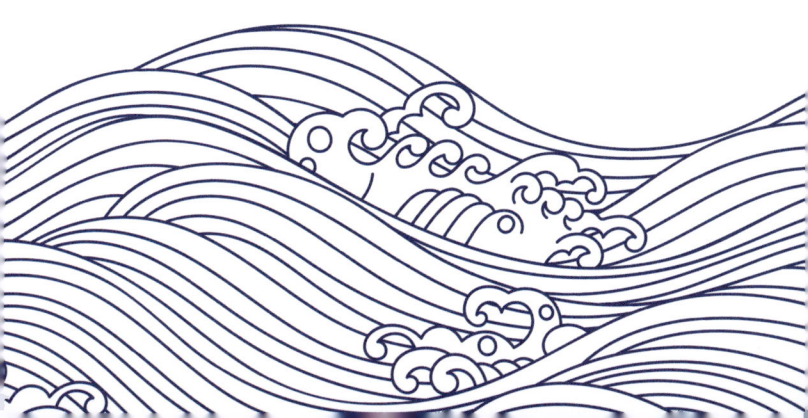

O
is for
Opportunity

The western world tends to promote anti-ageing as a way of tricking nature or turning back time. But reframing our older years as a continuous opportunity for learning and growth is a lot more interesting than trying to mask laugh lines. Instead of viewing ageing as something to fight against, it's helpful to think about it as a gathering of momentum – consider all the things your current self knows now that it didn't know five or ten years ago.

Multiply that into the future and you start to see how the wisdom of our years is a force for good.

Age is a number – and though we often fixate on our chronological age as a defining feature, there are other benchmarks. Did you know that your physiological age – how your body is ageing at a cellular level – can be different to your chronological age? Similarly, we can look at other markers, such as emotional age or social intelligence. Where physiological age is about quality not quantity, emotional and social agility often increase as we age. We become less volatile and more measured.

In many of the famed "blue zones", where most people live long and healthy lives, extended family life is the norm rather than the exception. In fact, people living in blue zones tend to prioritize multi-generational living with one generation caring for another. Great news for grandparents who care for their grandchildren and are therefore more likely to live longer.

Embrace the opportunities that come with age by creating positive affirmations.

1. Close your eyes and consider what fears you hold about ageing. Is it a loss of independence? Physical or mental decline? Write them all down.

....
....
....
....
....

2. Now, shift your mind to strengths you hold or have developed over the course of your life. Write down all you can think of here.

....
....
....
....
....

3. How could you use your strengths to reframe your fears from step one? For example: "I'm a source of wisdom and joy for my family and friends." "My mind and body are adapting gracefully as I age." Write your affirmations here.

P

is for
Pets

While the jury's still out on whether being a pet parent might actually make you live longer, there's firm evidence to support that it impacts overall happiness and well-being. For example, here's what the science says about dog ownership:

- Dogs provide emotional support. They're not called man's best friend for nothing! The loyal companionship of a dog can significantly reduce feelings of isolation.

Dogs also encourage exercise – it turns out we benefit from those daily walks as much as our four-legged friends do.

- Petting a dog lowers stress and blood pressure. Plus, they usually quite like it.
- Dogs provide routine and purpose. Our furry friends are totally dependent on us for food, water and care. Being their caregivers provides a sense of responsibility and meaning.
- Most dogs are social creatures. Dogs are natural conversation starters, especially with other dog owners. Plus, people love talking about their pets, too, so you'll never be at a loss for words.
- Dogs offer comfort and joy. They don't care if your hair is a bit messy or whether you've got a hole in your sock. They simply want to spend time with you.
- Dogs encourage playfulness. Whether it's a game of fetch or a random fit of the "zoomies", dogs are natural sources of fun.

You can make a dog's day with these homemade treats. No pooch of your own? Brighten the day of a neighbour's dog or, even better, take some to a local shelter.

Ingredients:
- 180 g oats
- 2 ripe bananas (medium)
- 120 g natural peanut butter

Method:
- Preheat the oven to 150°C.
- Line a baking sheet with parchment paper.
- Grind the oats in a blender or food processor.
- Add the bananas and peanut butter, continue mixing until a sticky dough is formed.
- Roll out onto a lightly floured surface and shape with a cookie cutter or cut into squares.
- Bake for 20 to 25 minutes, until brown on the edges and bottom.
- Cool before serving.

The truest, purest

love is the love that

comes from your dog.

Oprah Winfrey

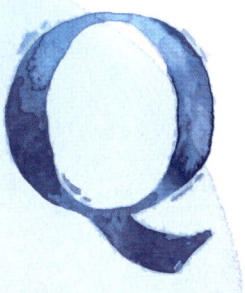

is for
Quality of Life

Longevity isn't just about a number, it's about the life in your years. Active ageing encourages a well-rounded approach to growing old, by engaging in activities that stimulate our minds, bodies, spirits and emotions.

Here are some helpful hints on active ageing:

💧 Stay connected – older adults who have close friends and family may live longer and reduce their risk of age-related depression.

- Think positive – staying positive about ageing can add seven and a half years to your life.
- Remain curious – intellectual engagement is just as important as physical activity when it comes to longevity. Read books on new and interesting subjects, listen to different types of music, do a jigsaw or learn a new language – all great ways to get the grey matter firing.
- Cultivate calm – stress is a killer. It can have a negative impact on almost every system of the body. Continuous, sustained stress can manifest into physical ailments or exacerbate existing weaknesses. As we age, we might come under different, perhaps unexpected, stressors from different daily routines. Having an outlet for stress relief is essential for active ageing.
- Stay engaged – participation in community or cultural events provides a sense of belonging and usefulness. Volunteering for local establishments or involvement in local civic groups provides a great sense of purpose and satisfaction.

Our quality of life is greatly enhanced when we fill our days with meaningful activities. We can identify where our passion and mission meet with this exercise. Write a list of the things you love doing, the things you're good at doing and what the world or your community needs. How might these align, so you can start living more purposefully?

What I love doing	What I'm good at	What the world needs

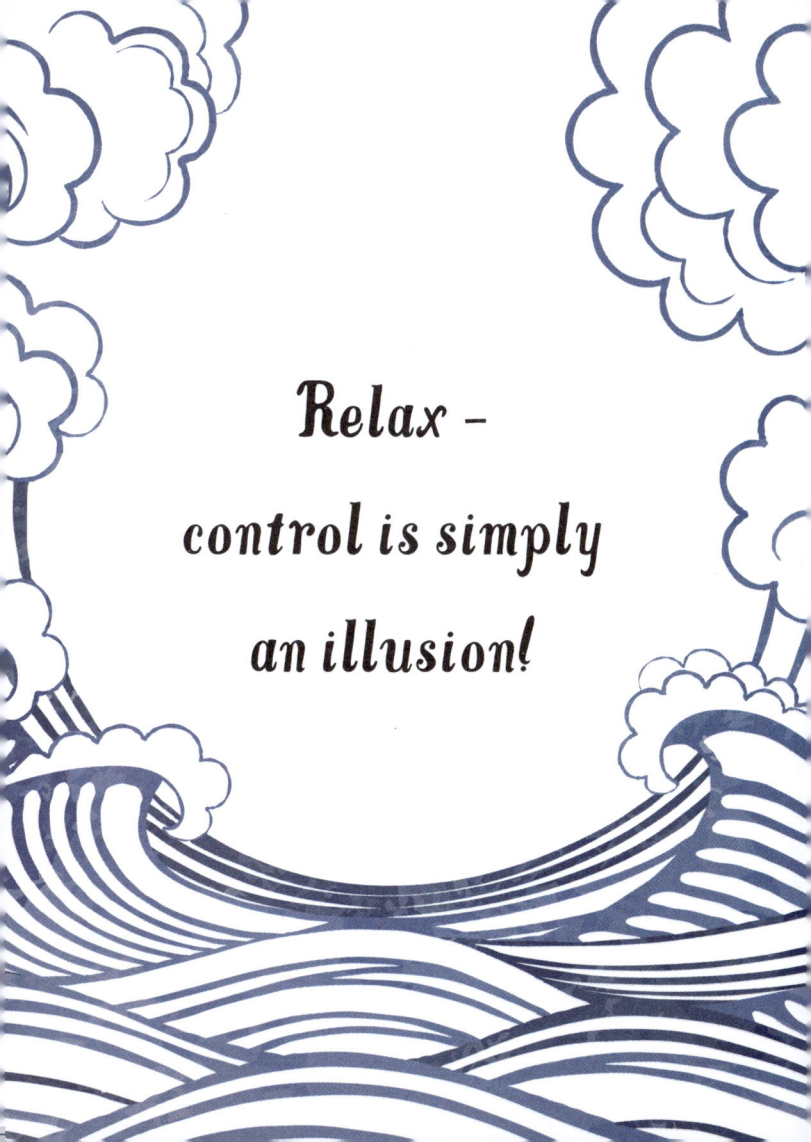

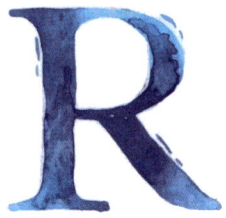

is for
Relaxation

The art of relaxation is one that very few of us have mastered. Our lifestyles tend to value movement over stillness and relaxation. Oftentimes, even our weekends and days off are packed with plans. While some activities we enjoy make us feel relaxed, that's different from relaxation as a state of being. True relaxation is a release of all effort – physical, mental and even emotional.

For many of us, relaxation is something that comes around occasionally, perhaps while on holiday or after a day of work and play. Unfortunately, this replenishment of energy is not true relaxation.

One route to an enhanced state of relaxation is through meditation and mindfulness practices. These are proven to promote longevity, by reducing stress and inflammation, and even improving gut health.

Ironically, achieving a state of relaxation can take effort. With all our roles and responsibilities, it might feel a bit indulgent to prioritize doing nothing. But sometimes, the busier we are, the more we need rest and relaxation, and the more we need to schedule downtime into our days and weeks. It might feel a bit uncomfortable at first, which is probably a strong indicator that it's working!

A body scan is a mindfulness technique that helps relax the mind and body. It can be done anywhere, either as a guided meditation or in your own time. As you scan the body from head to toe, you'll start to become aware of any sensations that are present in the body. Try not to engage with any feelings you may encounter. Simply note their presence. During the exercise, there's no need for any physical movement or deliberate relaxation of the body; simply move your awareness around the body from point to point.

1. Start by closing your eyes and taking three deep breaths in and out.
2. Bring your awareness to the top of your head, then to your forehead, eyes, eye sockets, ears, cheekbones, mouth and jaw.
3. Move your awareness down to your neck and throat, then to the tops of the shoulders.
4. Next, shift your focus to your upper arms, then elbows, lower arms, wrists, hands and fingers.
5. Bring awareness to your chest, ribcage, belly and lower back.

6. Move down to your hips and pelvis, then to your thighs, knees and kneecaps.

7. Finally, shift your awareness to your calves, shins, ankles, feet and right down to your toes.

8. Spend a few breaths being present and aware of your whole body, plus the space your body occupies.

9. When you're ready, slowly open your eyes, feeling relaxed and refreshed.

Use the space below to note down how you feel after doing this body-scan activity. See if you can spot any benefits after performing it for a few days.

....
....
....
....
....
....
....
....

Exercise is the key

not only to physical health

but to peace of mind.

Nelson Mandela

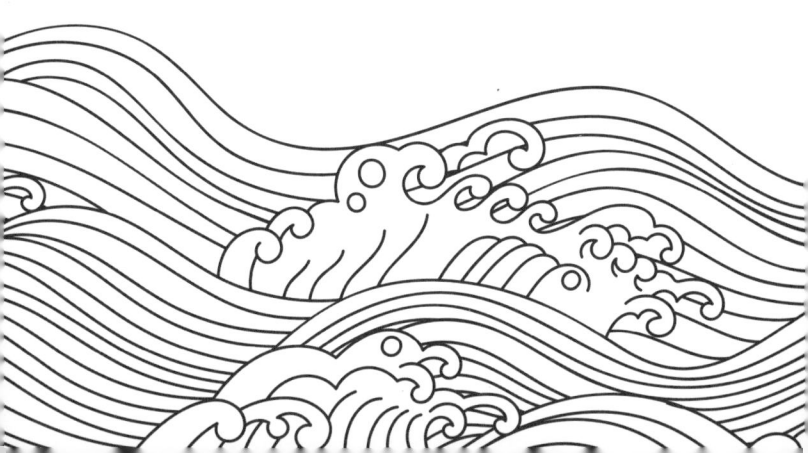

> The quality of life is determined by its activities.
>
> Aristotle

S

is for
Sleep

Is there anything more refreshing than a good night's sleep? Whether you are physically or mentally tired, the restorative powers of sleep can literally herald the dawn of a new day. But there's good news for the night owls out there – it turns out sleep patterns are more important than duration. In fact, irregular sleeping patterns can have an adverse effect on cardiac health, epigenetic ageing, mood and overall quality of life.

Sleep is our body's natural restoration time. Our bodies go into repair mode when we sleep, repairing muscle and tissue damage, and processing and storing memories. The space between our brain cells also increases when we sleep, allowing fluids in to flush away toxins. Circadian rhythms run on 24-hour cycles, balancing the systems of the body, including hormone regulation, digestion and body temperature. Interfering with the biological body clock can have a negative impact on how we look and feel, as well as on our mood and energy levels.

Lack of sleep can lead to multiple health complications, including higher blood pressure and blood sugar levels, increased belly fat and decreased brain function.

Do we naturally sleep less as we age? On average, older adults still need around 7 hours of sleep daily, but your sleep architecture may shift, making you sleepy earlier but wide awake at the crack of dawn. The key is consistency – keep to a regular sleep pattern to get the most out of your zzzs.

Try the 8-3-2-1-0 sleep rule. Track your progress over one week and make a note of how you feel each morning.

- 8: Don't consume caffeine within 8 hours of bedtime.
- 3: Don't consume food or alcohol in the 3 hours before bedtime.
- 2: Stop work at least 2 hours before bed.
- 1: Shut off all screens at least 1 hour before bed – no TV, mobiles or tablets.
- 0: Don't rely on the snooze button when the alarm goes off.

Use the tracker below for a week, to help you track your sleeping routine progress.

Sunday: 8☐ 3☐ 2☐ 1☐ 0☐

....

Monday: 8☐ 3☐ 2☐ 1☐ 0☐

....

Tuesday: 8☐ 3☐ 2☐ 1☐ 0☐

....

Wednesday: 8☐ 3☐ 2☐ 1☐ 0☐

....

Thursday: 8☐ 3☐ 2☐ 1☐ 0☐

....

Friday: 8☐ 3☐ 2☐ 1☐ 0☐

....

Saturday: 8☐ 3☐ 2☐ 1☐ 0☐

....

T

is for
Tai Chi

This ancient Chinese martial art is sometimes called "meditation in motion". It's a series of postures that are performed in a slow flow of continuous movement. Though it might look gentle, it has the potential to burn as many calories as conventional exercise. It's also been found to improve brain functions, such as memory and mental flexibility, faster than any other physical exercise.

While tai chi might be called meditation in motion, a growing body of evidence points to it acting as a kind of *medication* through motion. Some even go so far as to say it can be used as an adjunct treatment to conventional medicine, for the prevention and rehabilitation of injury and disease.

Tai chi differs from traditional exercise in a few significant ways. It links breath and movement, increasing that mind–body link and reducing stress. The movements are circular, promoting a natural fluidity in the body that builds strength and flexibility. At the same time, they are gentle on the joints, which are never fully flexed or bent throughout the series of postures. In traditional Chinese medicine, circular movements also boost your *qi*, or "vital energy".

Despite its soft approach, tai chi can also help with weight loss and contribute to better sleep for regular practitioners.

Weight shifting is a beginner-level warm-up that improves balance and coordination. It can be practised almost anywhere – try it close to a wall or chair for extra stability.

1. Start by standing tall, feet hip-width apart, weight evenly distributed across both feet.
2. Keep a soft bend in your knees.
3. Slowly shift your weight to your right leg, lifting your left foot slightly off the ground.
4. Hold for one slow breath in and out.
5. Return to the centre and repeat on the other side.
6. Repeat several times.

Weight shifting helps build strength and stability – great for preventing falls at any age.

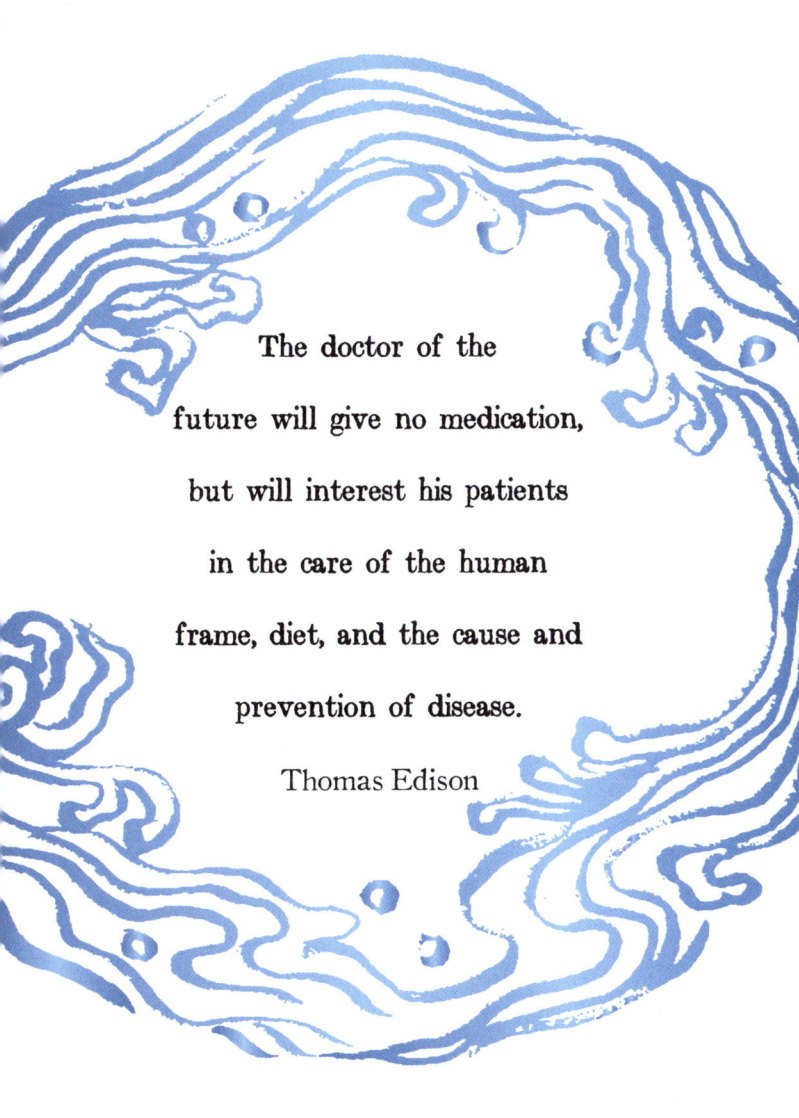

The doctor of the future will give no medication, but will interest his patients in the care of the human frame, diet, and the cause and prevention of disease.

Thomas Edison

U

is for
Unburden

Sometimes, we carry around unhelpful feelings that hold us back from reaching our full potential. Anger, regret, upset – things we wish we had said or done, or those we wish we hadn't. This unspent negative energy can take up a lot of headspace and influence our behaviour if we let it. Releasing these negative emotions can lighten our load and help us move into our later years with courage and conviction.

But how do we let go of the road not taken? First, it's about identifying our limiting beliefs. Listen for the "no" that comes up when you want to try something new. Statements such as, "I can't do that", or, "that's not for me", are telltale signs you might be touching on a limiting belief. Try challenging these thoughts – how would you feel if you tried it and it *did* work out? What do you know now that you didn't know back then, which makes you more likely to succeed?

Still not sure? Try writing things down. When you notice anger or upset flaring, ask yourself why. What's behind the anger? Are you scared? Worried? Unpacking your emotions can start to loosen years of learned negativity.

A releasing ceremony is a way to let go of unhelpful feelings in a supportive way. Releasing ceremonies can be done at any time, but symbolically you might want to align yours with the full moon, or the end of a season or year.

1. Grab some paper and a pen, and find a quiet, comfortable place.
2. Bring to mind any thoughts or emotions that are no longer serving you.
3. Write down everything you are ready to release.
4. Take a moment to acknowledge the lessons learned from each thing on the list.
5. Symbolically "release" the paper, by either burning it or tearing it up into pieces.
6. Close your eyes and visualize a pure white light entering your body, filling the space you have created with the release.

Every moment is a fresh beginning.

T. S. Eliot

V

is for
Visualization

Can you visualize a long and healthy future for yourself? There's good news if you can, as some studies have shown that people who believe they will be healthy in many years' time are more likely to achieve that outcome. Your mind and body is interconnected and, while diet and exercise are crucial for nurturing your physical body, you can enhance your overall well-being with the power of visualization. Learning to mentally map out your later life can influence your current behaviour and even help you achieve your desired outcomes.

How does visualization work? By creating a picture in your mind of your desired outcome, you fire up the neurons in your brain and almost trick it into thinking it's already true. Since your brain believes this is the direction of travel, it gets started figuring out the pathway to make it happen. Many athletes use visualization as a part of their practice and preparation. By seeing themselves achieving their goals – breaking that record or scoring the winning goal – they're able to turn these thoughts into reality.

Visualization can also be used as a "compare and contrast" tool. You can imagine the outcome of your current actions. Using this kind of "if… then…" logic can start to influence the decisions you make. So remember, if you can think it and believe it, you can achieve it!

Try this "future self" visualization. Close your eyes and imagine yourself in the future. You're strong, healthy and full of vitality. How do you interact with the world? How do you spend your time? With whom? How do you look after yourself?

Open your eyes and write down your vision.

....
....
....
....
....
....
....
....

Top tip

You can reinforce this visualization with a vision board. Using photos or words, create a collage that reflects your future self. Keep the collage somewhere that means you see it regularly.

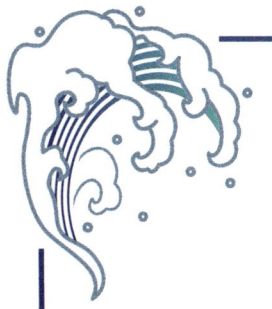

Manifest your perfect life through visualization and affirmation

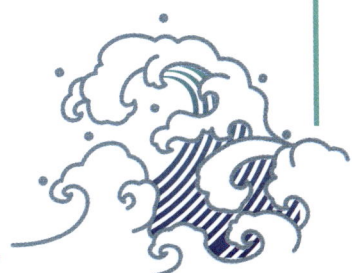

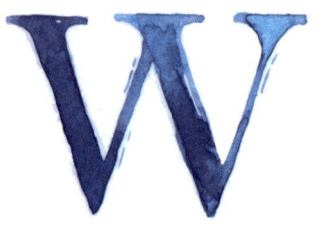

is for *Walking*

Sometimes overlooked due to its simplicity, a daily stroll is one of the most effective ways to extend your longevity. A regular brisk walk can help trim the waistline, lower blood pressure, lift mood, and strengthen bones and muscles. Women who walk for 7 or more hours a week have an added bonus of a 14 per cent reduction in risk of getting breast cancer than those who walk 3 or fewer hours per week. Walking 160 minutes per day can increase your lifespan by up to five years.

Walking faster, further and more frequently reaps extra benefits, but even short walks can help curb chocolate cravings and reduce your intake of sugary snacks. Walking helps you sleep better, particularly if you walk outside and are exposed to natural light. When we walk, we increase the flow of blood, oxygen and nutrients to the brain. One protein in particular, BDNF, stimulates the growth of new brain cells and connections.

Getting out for a daily walk can reduce your risk of depression, high blood pressure, type 2 diabetes and sleep apnoea. Walking can even save you money, as you'll spend less on petrol when you ditch the car and go by foot. Finally, walking is a great form of social exercise when done with a friend, in a group or with a four-legged companion.

To increase your daily steps, it's important to incorporate walking into your routine in small but manageable ways. Here are five ideas for increasing your daily step count:

- Take the stairs – choose the stairs over escalators or elevators wherever possible.
- Phone calls – when calling a friend or family member, choose to take a walk throughout the call.
- For errands – whenever possible, choose to walk to run any errands, be it going to a café or a quick run to the grocery store.
- Make a date of it – get a walking buddy, for regular walking catch-ups.
- Join the club – look for local walking clubs or join a charitable challenge, to add some additional incentive to your step count.

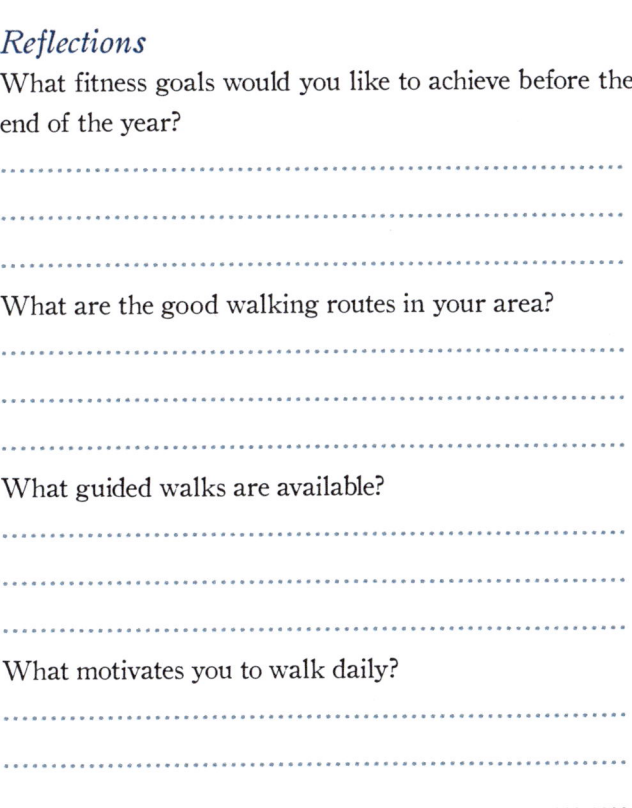

Reflections

What fitness goals would you like to achieve before the end of the year?

....

....

....

What are the good walking routes in your area?

....

....

....

What guided walks are available?

....

....

....

What motivates you to walk daily?

....

....

....

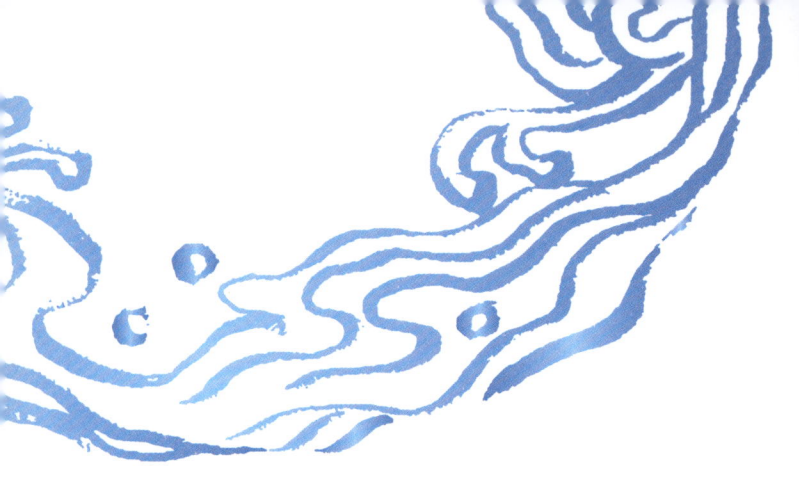

A journey of

a thousand miles begins

with a single step.

Lao Tzu

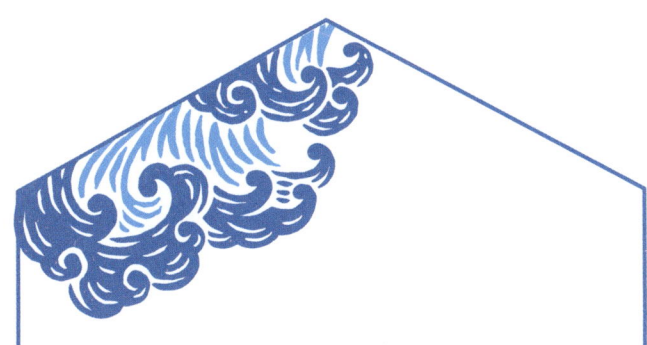

Engage in activities that nourish

and care for your body's well-being

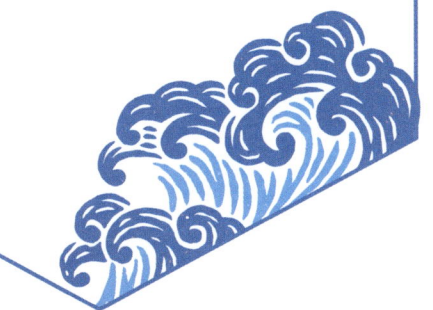

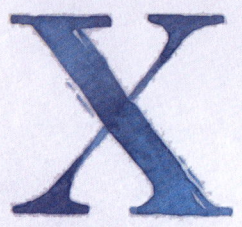

is for
XOXO

Loving relationships not only make us happier, but they also contribute to making us healthier. For men, in particular, it seems that stable relationships increase their health and decrease multiple risk factors. When bad things do happen, both men and women experience faster healing when they are supported in loving relationships.

The happily hitched also enjoy lower blood pressure than their single or unhappily matched friends. Marriage itself isn't a factor, however; cohabitating loving couples receive the same benefits. The stability of long-term loving relationships also decreases anxiety and eases stress. A problem shared is a problem halved when it comes to love, and we're less likely to suffer from depression when we feel emotionally connected to our partners. As we age, sometimes our world seems to get a bit smaller. Having that dependable person by your side can provide comfort and also give you courage to pursue new hobbies or adventures.

Perhaps more surprisingly, love can improve your gut health, too. Up to 80 per cent of your immune cells live in your gut, and feeling loved can nurture that microbiome, playing a crucial role in digestion.

Despite any duvet duels, being in a loving relationship also helps us sleep better, by reducing our stress and easing tension.

Try the "three and three" exercise with your partner or loved one. You'll each need a pen and paper. Start by sitting in a quiet place apart from each other. Think of three things you love about the person you're with and three things you don't love. Be honest but kind – think of this as an opportunity for growth. After a set time, come back together and alternate sharing your "three and three" list. Be sure to end on a positive note.

Three things I love about my partner/friend:

....

....

....

Three things I don't love about my partner/friend:

....

....

....

What I learned through this experience:

....

....

....

When we love, we always strive

to become better than we are.

When we strive to become

better than we are, everything

around us becomes better too.

Paulo Coelho

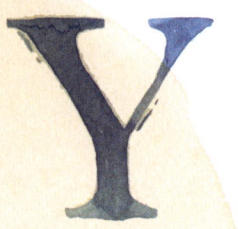

is for
Yoga

The ancient art of yoga has become a fixture in the western world for good reason – it's an enjoyable way to exercise with lots of extra benefits. Yoga is a mixture of movement and breath. It comes in many different forms, but even the gentlest practice can yield great rewards. Practising yoga can impact on various predictors of longevity, such as walking speed and leg strength. Yoga can also help improve balance, which is particularly important in our later years, as falls are a leading contributing factor to more serious illnesses.

Research shows that yoga may influence ageing at a cellular level. Regular yogis can reduce their metabolism to a state similar to that of hibernating animals. There's evidence that slowing down your breathing and heart rate can lead to increased lifespan. What's more, yoga can reduce blood pressure, blood fat levels, stress and anxiety.

Physically, yoga is an accessible form of exercise that focuses on keeping the spine flexible. There are five different types of movements recommended: forward folding, backward bending, side bending, twists and inversions – all which have physical benefits. While yoga helps increase flexibility and strength, many yogis will tell you it's not about touching your toes, but what you learn on the way down. Yoga is a way to get to know yourself physically and spiritually. Plus, the *savasana* (final resting pose) isn't too bad either.

Yoga is a way to explore movement and breath to make the body feel good. If you're practising yoga for the first time, be sure not to push your body too far, as you don't want to hurt yourself. To begin, try moving in a gentle and expansive way in cat/cow:

1. Start on all fours with a neutral (straight) spine.
2. Inhale, turning your tailbone up, dropping your belly down and looking up to the sky.
3. Exhale, turning your tailbone down, drawing your belly button to your spine and tucking your chin to your chest.
4. Repeat for five or six rounds.

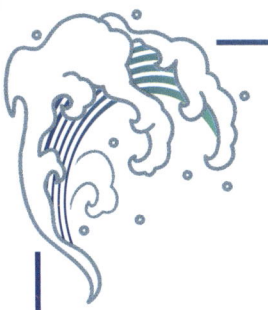

The art of practising yoga is all about the journey you take within yourself

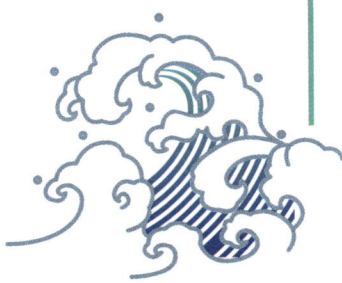

Z

is for
Zest

Don't fall into the trap of trying to be so healthy that you forget to have fun. Life is meant to be lived, not as a bystander, but as a fully fledged player. People who approach life with curiosity, joy and a sense of purpose maintain healthier lifestyles, both physically and mentally.

Scientific studies support the idea that a positive outlook can reduce the risk of cardiovascular disease, lower inflammation and enhance immune function. People with a zest for life are also more likely to stay socially engaged, pursue meaningful goals and remain physically active – all key predictors of a longer, healthier life. When life feels exciting and worth living, it's easier to make choices that support well-being, such as eating well, exercising and avoiding harmful habits.

In essence, zest for life isn't just a feel-good attitude, it's a powerful psychological asset that promotes vitality and longevity. Cultivating it through hobbies, relationships and purpose can significantly enhance both the quality and length of your life.

Be inspired: Betty Goedhart set a record when she became the oldest female flying trapeze artist at age 84. She was first fascinated by the sport as a child, but didn't start practising until she was 78 – proof positive that you're never too old to try something new!

Variety is the spice of life, and we all enjoy different things. Spend some time thinking about the things that really light you up inside, and write them all down on the zest wheel. Feel free to play around with different categories if the ones below don't resonate. See what aspects of your life are bringing you that extra joy and perhaps find ways either to spend more time on those activities or add zest to the areas that need boosting.

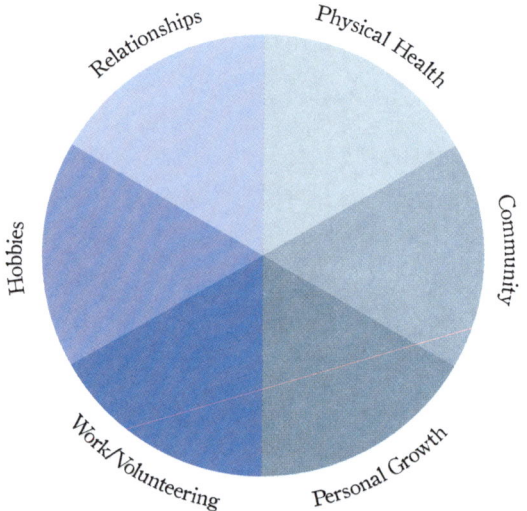

I don't believe people are looking for the meaning of life as much as they are looking for the experience of being alive.

Joseph Campbell

Conclusion

The A–Z of Longevity underscores a powerful truth: while our genes lay the foundation, our daily choices shape the life we live, as well as the length and quality of that life. Longevity doesn't hinge solely on luck or biology, but is linked to intention, attention and gentle consistency.

Throughout this book, we've explored the small, meaningful habits that can have a big impact over time. Moving your body regularly, fostering strong connections with others, eating nourishing foods, filling your days with purpose and prioritizing restorative sleep – none of these are difficult or dramatic, but they *are* deeply powerful. Practised consistently, they form pillars of lasting vitality and well-being.

Longevity isn't about chasing eternal youth or perfection. It's about cultivating the conditions for a long, fulfilling life, rich with meaning, energy and joy. Each letter of this A–Z has offered a reminder that what we do today shapes the life we'll enjoy tomorrow.

So, take what resonates and begin wherever you are. Let movement be your medicine, connection your comfort, food your fuel and sleep your sanctuary. Return to these basics often, building upon the foundation for a long and happy life.

May this book serve not as an end, but as a beginning – a gentle companion that reminds you of your power to shape your future, one simple, life-affirming choice at a time.

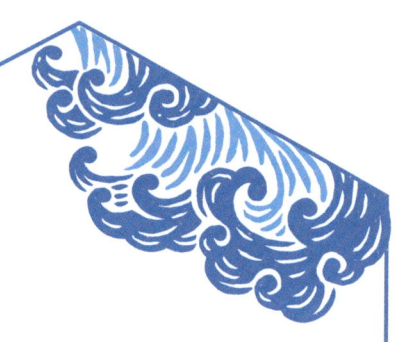

Surround yourself with people who encourage and support healthy choices

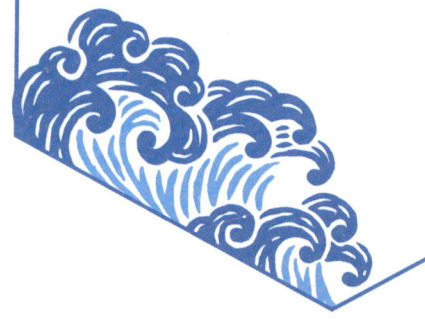

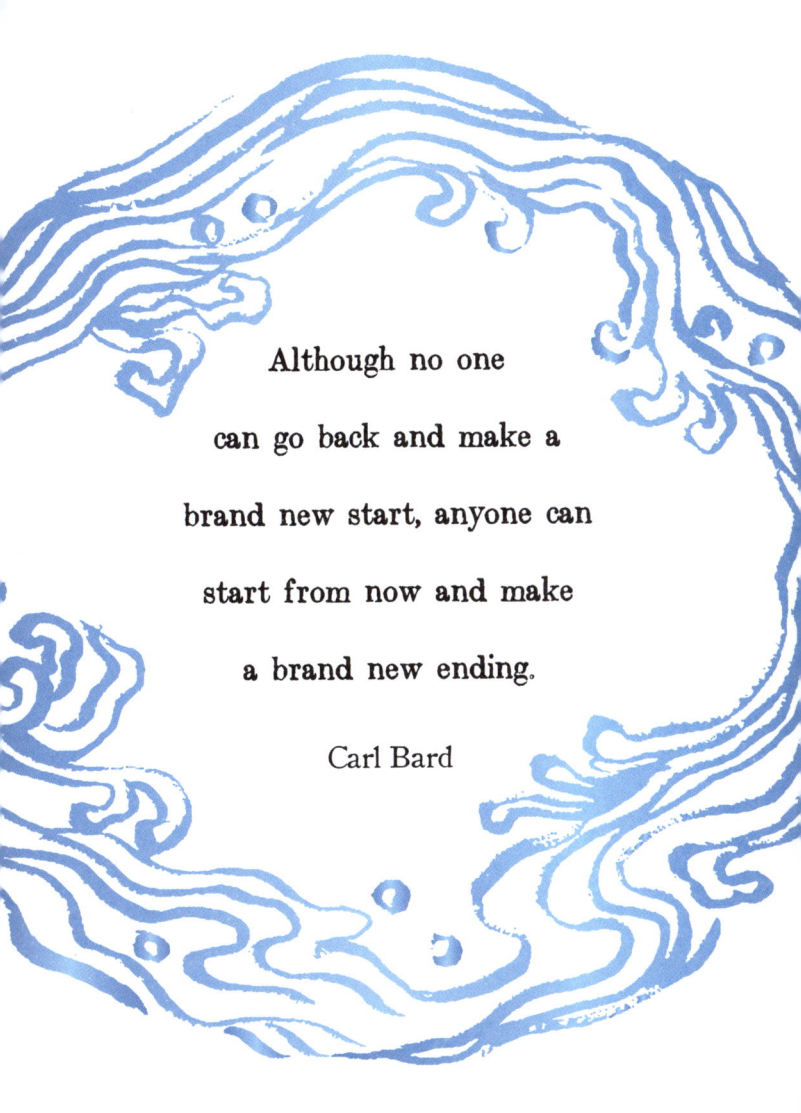

Although no one can go back and make a brand new start, anyone can start from now and make a brand new ending.

Carl Bard

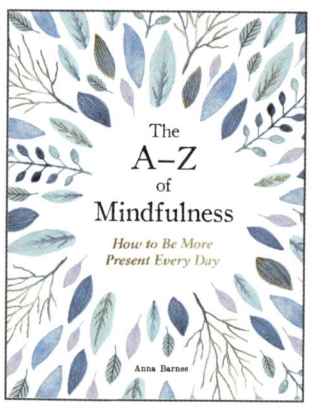

The A–Z of Mindfulness
Anna Barnes
ISBN: 978-1-78783-273-2
Hardback

Squeeze every drop out of each moment and live life to the full by discovering the art of mindfulness. Learn new ways to connect with yourself and the world around you and reignite a sense of wonder in the everyday with this practical ABC of illustrated tips for mindful living.

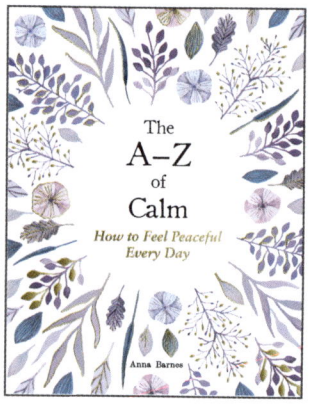

The A–Z of Calm
Anna Barnes
ISBN: 978-1-83799-008-5
Hardback

Go on a journey through the pages of *The A–Z of Calm* to discover an array of mindful and meditative exercises that will help you locate your inner peace. With a helpful tip for every letter of the alphabet, learn how to pinpoint your stress triggers and discover how you can find a pocket of calm in our hectic modern-day society.

Image Credits

pp. 3, 28, 53, 86 © i176/Shutterstock.com; pattern fill © Rolau Elena/Shutterstock.com

pp. 4, 5, 8, 9, 14, 18, 22, 26, 27, 29, 32, 36, 40, 44, 48, 52, 56, 57, 59, 62, 66, 67, 72, 73, 76, 77, 80, 84, 85, 90, 94, 98, 102, 106, 107, 112, 113, 116, 120, 122, 123 water droplets © Rolau Elena/Shutterstock.com

Letter heads throughout © anna42f/Shutterstock.com

Spots throughout © Alena Tselesh/Shutterstock.com

pp. 10, 37, 63, 87, 99 textured background (all colours) © Rolau Elena/Shutterstock.com

pp. 11, 45, 58, 90, 109, 124 blue waves © Tirta Sudibya/Shutterstock.com

pp. 15, 68, 103, 117 white waves © PSAROV SERHII/Shutterstock.com

pp. 19, 49, 121 water droplets (in circle) © Rolau Elena/Shutterstock.com

pp. 23, 69, 81 sea © TWINS DESIGN STUDIO/Shutterstock.com

pp. 33, 41, 95, 108, 125 water arc © queso/Shutterstock.com

p. 48 jar © freshcare/Shutterstock.com

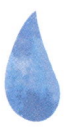

Have you enjoyed this book?
If so, why not write a review on your favourite website?

If you're interested in finding out more about our books, find us on Facebook at **Summersdale Publishers,** on Twitter/X at @**Summersdale** and on Instagram, TikTok and Bluesky at @*summersdale.books* and get in touch. We'd love to hear from you!

Thanks very much for buying this Summersdale book.

www.summersdale.com

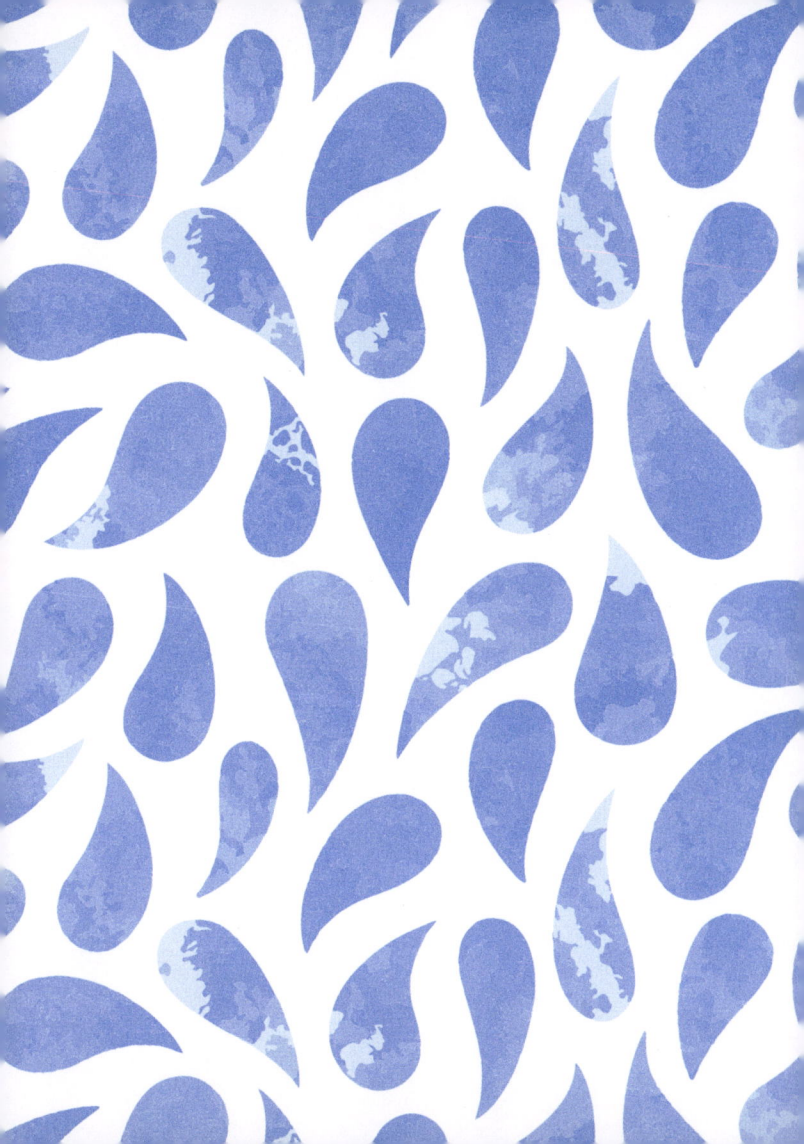

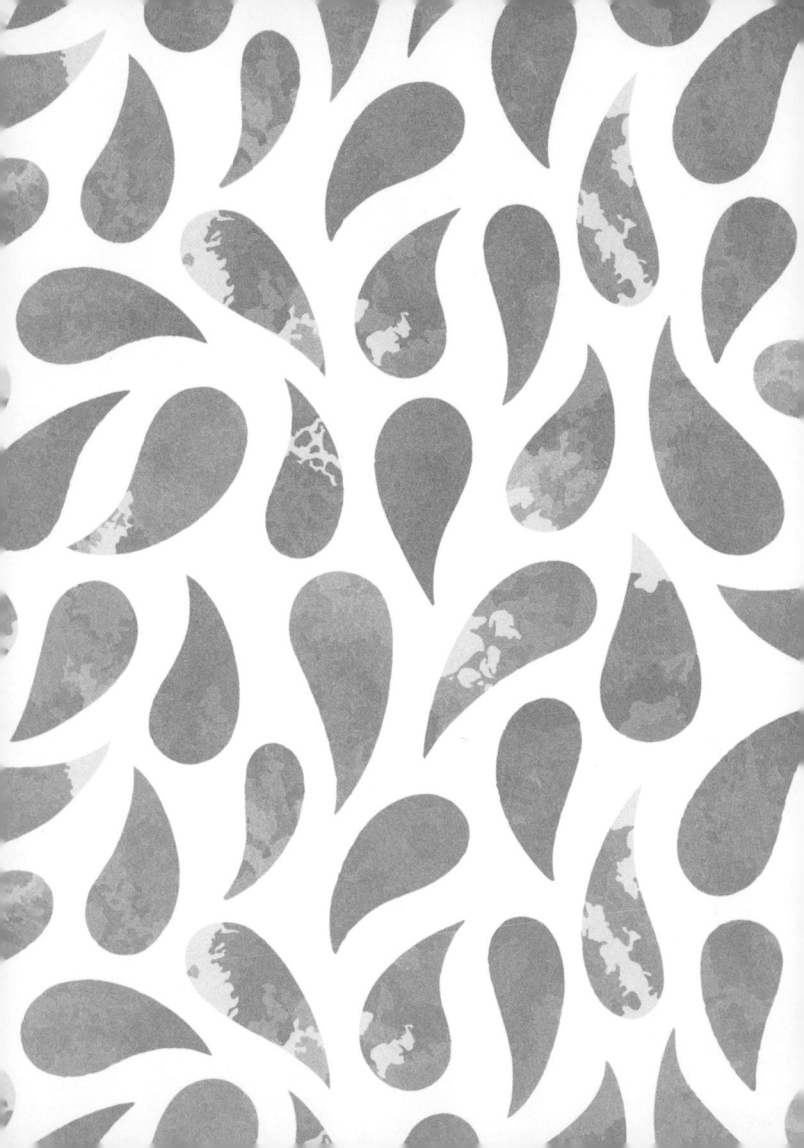